S
Meta
Speed Up your Metabolism
and Lose Weight Quickly
Steven Ballinger

Super Fast
Metabolism Diet

Super Charge Metabolism
and Lose Weight Quickly

Sierra Gillfiane

Legal Disclaimer

Introduction

The desire to lose weight and stay fit is becoming more and more difficult to satisfy. After all, most restaurants have increased their portion sizes to the point where one entree often has an entire day's worth of calories.

If you go to McDonald's and order a Happy Meal for your child, the cheeseburger inside used to be the cheeseburger that adults would order. It's not just fast food places, though. The vast majority of eateries are using bigger and bigger plates.

At the same time, the modern lifestyle is becoming less and less active. More and more jobs involve expertise with computers in some form or fashion. This means that more people are spending more of their work day seated at a chair, staring at a screen.

When people come home from work, many of their entertainment forms (television, surfing the Net, playing video games) involve doing some more sitting. Getting outside and being active are pursuits that are becoming an endangered species.

The good news is that finding ways to manage your weight and keep it at the level you want is not impossible. It starts with finding ways to boost the rate at which your body burns the fuel you put into it - in other words, the rate of your metabolism. When it comes to whether you lose or gain weight, there is just one simple formula: if you eat more calories than you burn through activity, you will gain weight. If you burn more calories than you eat, then you will lose weight. Finding ways to speed up your metabolism will help you come out on the right side of this equation more often than not.

This book contains a guide to the types of food you should eat and types of food you should avoid. There are recipes, exercises and other tips to help you take charge of your metabolism. The advice in this book can help you change your life for the better. So let's get started!

1: Understanding Your Own Unique Metabolism

If you are trying to lose weight, you may wonder about how your metabolism works, particularly when you do not think you are losing weight as quickly as you should.

In this chapter, we will discuss some reasons why some people's metabolisms are slower than others, as well as some tips you can use to speed things up.

For most people, when you start to lose weight, the pounds come off easily - at least the first five or even ten. A lot of this is excess water that you were carrying around; many people who cut back on their consumption also cut back on what they are drinking, and the body sheds water as a result. However, they then hit a plateau, and one of the first scapegoats for this is their slow metabolisms.

The technical meaning of metabolism has to do with the way that the human body uses energy, through such processes as muscular function, food digestion and even breathing.

All of the body's processes require energy to take place. If you think about each one of your cell as a small engine, needing fuel to operate, then you have a sense of how the metabolism functions.

The key term here is metabolic rate, or the rate at which your body burns up energy. BMR (basal metabolic rate) refers to the speed at which you use up your calories. If you have a slow metabolism and have a difficult time losing weight, you may have a more efficient method for burning calories, because you burn them more slowly and turn more of them into fat to use later.

This came in handy back when people lived by subsistence farming. People who burned calories more slowly were more likely to survive, particularly if they did not know where their next meal was coming from. People who were on the larger side were considered more attractive, first because they had the means to afford more food, and second because they had a higher probability of living through times of famine. Those who burned calories more efficiently were actually at a greater risk of starving to death.

In modern society, those who burn calories more efficiently end up having more of a weight problem. In most developed world, access to food is not a problem, and most occupations involve a sedentary lifestyle.

This means that people who lived in earlier centuries that were deemed healthy are now considered obese. Those who burn calories faster actually operate with a lower level of metabolic efficiency.

Scientists are still looking into the factors that help some people burn energy more quickly than others, but genetics can definitely have an effect in your metabolic rate.

Some studies have looked at familial trends over the course of generations and have found that it appears possible to inherit a particular body type, which means that we may be born with our metabolisms already established, at least within a particular range.

There are other factors that can influence your basal metabolic rate as well. If you do not get much exercise over the course of your day, because your job primarily involves sitting in front of a computer or at a desk, and because the majority of your leisure time is spent sitting and watching television or surfing the web, you can end up with a lower BMR. Studies show that lower levels of physical activity appear to have a correlation with slower metabolisms.

There are medical conditions that have an influence on metabolic rate as well. Hypothyroidism refers to a condition in which your body does not produce the right amount of thyroid hormone.

As a result, your metabolism works more slowly, and you have a greater likelihood of gaining weight than the rest of the population. Hyperthyroidism refers to the opposite situation: your body produces more thyroid hormone than you need. As a result, your body burns calories more quickly, and you can end up losing weight that you wanted to keep.

Both of these conditions are treatable through prescription drugs; *methimazole* and *radioactive iodine* are both used to slow down the metabolism for people suffering from hyperthyroidism. People who are hypothyroid generally receive treatment with a replacement hormone.

Another way you can increase your metabolic rate is through physical activity. Walking, running and other forms of aerobic exercise help you to burn more calories while you are doing them, but they can also boost your energy consumption rate while you are resting later on. Also, if you add muscle mass as a result of strength training, you can also boost your basal metabolic rate.

Sleep is another factor that influences your metabolism. If you're not getting enough sleep, your appetite can go up along with your resistance to insulin. This is a double whammy, because you're eating more food, but the hormone that helps you convert sugar into energy (insulin) is present in smaller amounts.

You are at risk of developing both diabetes and obesity in this situation. To keep this from happening, try to get between seven and nine hours per night for sleep.

There is actually a way to calculate your metabolic rate using an online calculator. If you enter your age, height, weight and gender, these devices can figure out how many calories your body burns per day. This is a rough estimate, of course; to get a precise answer, you often have to sleep in a testing facility and have it measured right when you wake up. The general principles that govern the calculator are as follows:

- The shorter you are, the lower your metabolism. The less you weigh, the lower your metabolism. Why? Because motion takes less energy.

- The older you are, the lower your metabolism. As time goes by, we need more and more exercise to burn calories at the same rate, because our metabolic engines do slow down. As a result, we need to cut back on what we eat and add to the amount of exercise we do. These changes will help keep metabolic rate as high as possible.

2: Foods That Will Speed Up Your Metabolism

There is no quick shortcut to the sort of weight loss that will last over the long haul. While there are some crash diets that you can use to lose weight quickly, as soon as you stop that restrictive (and often unhealthy) dietary regimen, the weight will come back.

However, there are some tweaks you can make to your diet if you want to boost your metabolism and make your body burn calories at a faster rate of speed. Obviously, you want to exercise regularly and make sure you get seven or more hours of sleep each night. However, adding the foods on this list will also get you where you want to go in terms of a speedier metabolism. Take this with you when you go to the grocery store.

1. *Broccoli*

Yes, there's a reason why your mom wanted you to get plenty of this vegetable in your diet. Broccoli has a lot of calcium (which has been shown to reduce weight). Broccoli also has a ton of Vitamins A, K and C. Vitamin C cuts the amount of cortisol in your system, which means you are not going to amass as much belly fat, and it also helps your body produce carnitine, which helps your system turn fat into fuel. In addition, broccoli is chock full of dietary fiber, folate and antioxidants. Not only will you be cutting fat, you will also be removing unwanted gunk from your digestive system.

1. *Purified Water*

You're right - water isn't TECHNICALLY a food. However, water does boost your metabolism, and it's best to drink water that is pure of all unwanted substances. A study in Germany discovered that you can speed up the fat burning process by drinking water. Water also keeps your appetite lower naturally.

1. *Foods that have a lot of Omega 3 fatty acids*

You want to have some fat in your diet if you're going to have a high revving metabolism. However, not all fats are the same; those that are high in Omega 3 fatty acids are actually good for your heart, as they contain the HDL or "good" cholesterol.

These acids cut down on the amount of leptin that your body produces. Leptin is a chemical that acts to slow down the metabolism; rodent studies at the University Wisconsin found that lower leptin levels led to higher metabolic rates.

Where can you find foods that are high in Omega 3 fatty acids? Check the labeling on butter and margarine products. However, some natural foods are walnuts, avocados and fish like salmon. A study from the Mayo Clinic analyzed the health of African tribes who consume a lot of fish. Their leptin levels were almost five times lower than the tribes that did not have access to fish. Adding these fatty acids to your diet is a must in a number of areas, but also for boosting your metabolism.

1. *Citrus Fruits*

Grapefruit, oranges, tangerines and other similar fruits have shown in studies that they spur the burning of fat while keeping the body's metabolism running high. The exact reason for the connection remains unclear, but it could be connected to the high levels of Vitamin C, which cuts the presence of cortisol as well as the spiking of insulin that can happen after a high-sugar meal.

1. *Foods with calcium*

A research study compared people who were taking in 1,200 or more milligrams of calcium each day with those who were not getting enough calcium. The result was that people at the higher calcium intake level lost almost twice as much weight as those with insufficient calcium. You can take calcium supplements to help with this, but if you are not a big fan of dairy foods, adding broccoli to your diet also adds to the calcium you are taking in.

1. Soups

If you start your meal with a bowl of soup, studies show that your subsequent eating will show a reduction in appetite. Combining soup with your meal speeds up your metabolism and helps your body burn fat. Make sure that your soup is based in broth, though, rather than cream.

1. Green Tea

Again, this isn't quite a food, but the extract in green tea has been shown, in numerous studies, to give your metabolism an increase. There are also some other benefits for your health, such as a wealth of antioxidants that can fight free radicals. These are molecules that get into your bloodstream through toxins in the environment and contribute to the aging process, as well as to disease.

1. Pears and apples

Both of these fruits have been shown to rev up the metabolism and increase weight loss. A study in Brazil showed that women who ate three small pears or apples each day lost significantly more weight than women who did not. Both of these fruits are generally available year-round, and they are generally inexpensive. Don't substitute canned pears (especially in that sugary syrup) or applesauce - you won't get the same benefit, because the raw fruits have more fiber.

1. *Spices*

The more pungent the spice, generally the higher a spice will rev your metabolism. Cinnamon, garlic, cayenne pepper, black pepper, powdered onion, ginger and mustard seeds are all flavors you can add to your diet in order to boost your metabolism. If you incorporate these spices into your diet, you can burn as many as 1,000 calories more each day, according to a Canadian research study.

1. *Hot Peppers*

Cayenne, habanero, jalapeno and other hot peppers give your circulation and metabolism a jump start. These foods not only make your metabolism run higher, but they also reduce cravings for food.

This comes from the capsaicin in the peppers; this substance sharpens the response of pain receptors in your body, sending your circulation and metabolism up. Have you ever eaten jalapenos and started sweating intensely? Then you know how this process works.

Consuming these peppers can make your metabolism run as much as 25 percent higher for as long as three hours after the meal.

Use these foods as part of your arsenal aimed at making your metabolism run higher. You'll feel better, and you'll start to see weight loss results sooner.

3: 10 Things You Can do to Lose weight

If you have a significant amount of weight to lose, it is tempting to go for crash diets and programs that offer a dramatic result in a short amount of time. This is why programs like the grapefruit diet, the Atkins diet, the South Beach diet, the apple diet, the cabbage diet, and the honey and lemon juice diet have all come and gone.

While elements of all of those programs have some validity, the bottom line is that there is only one way to get long term weight loss: commit to a lifestyle of diet and exercise that burns more calories than you take in. If you can do that, you will lose weight, and the weight will stay off. Here is a list of 10 things you can do to lose weight.

1. *Commit to a regular exercise program*

This doesn't mean you have to train for the next Boston Marathon. It does mean that you need to commit to exercising between 30 and 60 minutes a day, at least five days a week. If you choose five sessions, three of them should focus on cardio work, and two should focus on strength training. That combination will help you turn your body into a more efficient consumer of calories.

1. *Keep your exercise program diverse*

If you jog three miles a day, five days a week, at first you will notice some positive results. You'll drop a little weight, and you'll gain some toning in your legs. However, you will only be working a small percentage of your body's muscles.

After a while, your body will adjust to the workout routine it is used to so that it doesn't actually burn as many calories - your body will become more efficient. This is why you need to keep your body guessing by lifting weights, doing long and steady cardio, as well as shorter bursts of interval cardio workouts.

1.   *Keep a can of almonds in the car*

This will also work with walnuts and peanuts, but not with cashews, as the fat content is significantly higher. Many times, we head through the drive thru when we are hungry instead of finding something healthy to eat, and we end up with a bag of fries and a burger.

This counteracts all of the positive effects we want to produce with this program. Instead, reach into the console and eat a handful of nuts. The protein will be more filling than a bag of fries.

1.   *Give yourself a break now and then*

Is it ok to eat a small bowl of ice cream now and then? Absolutely. The rule of thumb is to follow your dietary rules 90 percent of the time. The closer you get to 100 percent, the more likely you are to have a major relapse and get into some binge eating. And when you do give yourself a treat, give yourself the permission to enjoy it.

If you make yourself feel guilty about it, you won't get any pleasure, and the stress may send you back to that same freezer later that night.

1.   *Tell a friend what you're doing*

If you're trying to lose weight, don't try alone. It's really hard to stay committed to a positive regimen of change, because even your body will be fighting against you. It's used to that high-carb, high fat diet, and it doesn't want to change. Having a friend keeping you on the right path will give you an extra line of defense when temptation to skip a workout or order fries instead of a salad hits.

1. *Throw all of the fat out of the refrigerator*

Ultimately, you want to teach your body to turn fat into fuel, instead of relying on sugar/glucose for energy. If you can train your body correctly, then your metabolism will operate more efficiently. So let yourself order some salmon or some lean beef. The Omega-3 fatty acids in those protein sources are good for your heart.

1. *Live off 100-calorie snack packs*

Some people radically alter their diet to the point where they eat their food in 100-calorie increments. They think that if they manage their lifestyle that way, it will be easier to keep control over the calories they consume.

While these snacks make a good weapon on those days when you just need an infusion of something sweet, they are not a viable food option for you. Focus on eating a balanced diet with mostly proteins and vegetables if you want to see optimal results.

1. *Keep telling yourself "one last pizza."*

The best day to begin your new regimen of change is today, not tomorrow. It's easy to tell yourself that you will make your first trip to the gym tomorrow, or that you will empty all of the Ho-Hos out of the pantry tomorrow. Instead, do it today. Seeing the fruits of your positive change will build the right kind of habits going forward, and it will make long term weight loss easier to attain.

1. *Don't beat yourself up when you slip*

For many people, overeating is a defense mechanism for stress. The purpose of this new program is to help you feel better and enjoy a healthier life. If you are dining out and decided to order strawberry shortcake for dessert when you've already had your treat this week, don't be hard on yourself emotionally.

Instead, make sure you get to the gym the next morning like you planned, and add some time on the treadmill. You'll feel better, because you'll be managing your life the way you want to.

1. Never Give up

You're feeling better, your clothes are a little looser, and so you think that it's time to dial back your effort. The first 10 pounds may come off easily because they consist mostly of water your body has stored up over time.

If you go back to your old habits after dropping those 10 pounds, you're going to see them come back - and maybe even bring back five or ten pounds more with them. You are committing to a new way of life, and you can do it. Never give up!

4: Foods and Habits to Avoid When Losing Weight

When it comes to losing a significant amount of weight, there are some lifestyle decisions that you simply have to accept. The days of eating dinner out of a fast food bag are over, unless you are planning on ordering something grilled or a salad - and those things generally taste much better from other restaurants.

The days of spending all of your leisure time in front of your television or your computer are over, because losing weight means committing to regular exercise. These are all positive outcomes, but changing habits can be difficult. Here is a list of some foods and other habits that you must eliminate from your life if you want a large-scale weight loss that will last.

1. *Get rid of the soda*

Even if you're drinking diet soda, it's time to replace it with water. The benefits of water over sugary sodas are obvious. If you replace a 20-ounce bottle of sugary soda with one of water each day, you would lose 35 pounds over the course of a year. With diet soda, studies show that drinking them leads you to take in more calories, perhaps because the fact that you're drinking something that tastes reasonably sweet without any calories leads you to think that you deserve other treats, and so you overeat.

1. *Manage or eliminate your alcohol consumption*

Alcohol is refined fruit juice. This means that it is mostly concentrated sugar. So when you drink alcohol, you are adding empty calories to your daily consumption with no nutritional benefit. So instead of drinking down those sugars late at night so they can turn to fat in your system, put the liquor down instead.

1. Shop the outer aisles of the grocery store

Produce, meats, fish and dairy generally make up the foods that goes around the outside of your grocery store. These are the most natural foods you will find in the store. Everything in the inner aisles (pasta, processed foods, popcorn, candy, cakes, and cookies) contains refined sugars. What's more insidious is that the more you consume these foods, the more you want them. Sticking to natural foods as much as possible will supercharge your diet.

1. Avoid anything with "Multigrain" on the label

This sounds like a baked product that has more dietary fiber in it. However, there is no regulatory definition for what comprises a multigrain product. As a result, many manufacturers simply stuff a bunch of processed carbs into a package and slap that word on the label, knowing that many well-intentioned dieters will buy it. The words "Whole Grain," on the other hand, do have a specific meaning, and that includes a healthy dose of dietary fiber.

1. Slow down when you're at the dinner table

Unless you are entering a pizza eating contest, you don't get any points for finishing your meal before everyone else at the table. The problem is that our hectic lives force us to shoehorn meals into small amounts of time. This starts in school, when we generally have just a half hour to leave class, get in line, get our food, find a table, eat, put our trash away, and then hurry to class.

In the workplace, lunches are often just as hurried if they do not turn into another opportunity to get work done. For your lifestyle to change, it is important to understand that meals are something to enjoy and to savor. This will give you a sense of being full before you overeat.

1. Eat breakfast

You might think that you're doing yourself a caloric favor by skipping breakfast. The research shows, though, that people who eat breakfast weigh less than people who skip it. Even if you skip out on this first meal, you are still likely to eat more calories over the whole day.

Begin your day with a breakfast that is healthy, containing both fiber and protein. An apple or a grapefruit half, along with a slice of whole grain toast and a scrambled egg combine for fewer than 300 calories, but you'll still stay full until it's time to eat lunch.

1. Refuse to surrender to restaurant size portions

When you go out to lunch or dinner, you are often served twice as many calories as you need. Restaurants have become accustomed to serving customers as much as they can eat instead of sticking with sensible portion sizes.

When the restaurant offers it, order the smaller portion of a meal. If not, ask the server to box up half of your entree to go. That way, you get a portion with a normal size without the temptation to keep on eating.

1. Stay away from unhealthy toppings and other add-ons

One of the more popular things to add to hamburgers is bacon. There is already a lot of beef on that bun, but the server still wants to sell you some bacon on top of it. Bacon is delicious, so the temptation is to go ahead and add it.

However, you're also adding unnecessary fat and salt. Creamy dressings and cheeses are also add-ons that radically change the nutritional content of the food that you eat. Check the calorie count (especially at fast food restaurants) as the chicken products and salads often have ingredients that drive the calorie number higher than burgers.

1. *Stop eating for the sake of eating*

So you're sitting in front of one of your favorite movies with a huge bowl of popcorn on the coffee table. You're reading a treasured novel with a bowl of Cheetos next to your hand. You're eating without really thinking about it, and without being hungry.

The outcome is more inches on your waistline without an improvement in nutritional content. Want a snack? Grab a bowl of baby carrots, or an apple, or a handful of nuts. You'll get full faster, and your waistline will thank you. Eliminating these habits will help you get the weight loss results you want.

5: High Metabolism Boosting Workout

There are two components to the equation of losing weight: diet and exercise. The dietary changes that you will have to make to lose weight may be numerous, but if you add an exercise program to your list of changes, you will find that weight loss comes much more easily.

Various exercise plans will give you different results as far as metabolic rate and dropped pounds. If you follow the principles in this plan, you will torch the calories as they come in, and you will notice fat vanishing with each passing week.

Embrace strength training

When you lift weights, you're not just increasing your metabolism during the workout. Studies show that your metabolism will stay 25 percent above normal rate for as long as 15 hours after you finish a strength training session at high intensity. If you make a habit of regular weight training, your metabolic engine will run at a higher rate on a consistent basis.

This workout focuses on using a slower process of lowering the weights, making all of your muscles work harder (leading to a higher caloric burn). With each rep, you pick up the weight over the count of two and then count to eight as you (much more slowly) bring the weight back down. If you can work in three workouts a week, you'll love your body and your metabolism.

Warm up

For four minutes, perform any sort of cardio at moderate intensity; this could include cycling, a stair climber, jogging, or an exercise machine. Then, alternate one strength exercise with three more minutes of cardio. Exercises like jogging in place, stepping up and down from a step bench, or jumping rope will allow you to do this without having to traipse all over the gym. Once the last weight exercise is done, cool down with four more minutes of cardio at moderate intensity.

The diagonal extension

This exercise targets your core, shoulders, outer thighs and quads. Pick up a five-pound dumbbell in your right hand. Hold it at shoulder height with your elbow bent keeping your palm facing down.

Lift your left foot a couple of inches out and to the side, keeping toes down to the floor while raising your heel. Then elevate your left knee up to your hip height, and lower the right arm across the body at a diagonal to a point outside your left knee. Hold for a count of 1, and then lift the arm and lower the leg within eight counts to begin. Carry this out 8-12 times; change to the other side and repeat.

The bridge fly

This exercise targets your shoulders, triceps, core, chest and hamstrings. Lie down on the floor, on your back, bending your knees, keeping your feet the same width as your hips, with a 12 pound dumbbell in each hand.

Extend the arms up above your shoulders, keeping your palms looking inward. Then pick up your glutes and lower back from up off the floor. Bend your elbows, lowering your arms over the course of eight slow counts. When your upper arm just barely contacts the floor, push back up in two counts.

Suspended Bridge

This exercise targets your triceps, shoulders, biceps, glutes, hamstrings, and core. Basically, it's you dangling from the edge of an exercise ball, your feet atop the ball and your hands underneath you.

Put your heels on the ball, and then set your hands on the floor, palms down. Point your fingertips toward your feet. Then, tighten your abdominal muscles and push your hips up from the floor.

Roll the ball ahead, keeping your chin forward and your head up. Hold this for one count, pushing your chest up toward the ceiling while all this is taking place.

Balance Lift

Pick up a five-pound dumbbell, keeping your palm facing the area behind you. Lean a bit ahead on your feet, lifting that left foot about half a foot up from the floor. Put your right hand on your hip, keeping your abs engaged. With that left leg still in the air, lift your left arm straight over your head, above the shoulder. Lower your back to the starting point in the count of 8. Make your goal 8 reps, and then change sides.

Roll and Curl

This exercise targets your glutes, thighs, quads, core, and biceps. Bend your left knee while standing, and put your left toe on a stability ball. Hold a ten-pound dumbbell in each hand. Now, straighten the left leg toward the side, moving the ball away from you.

While you are moving the ball, also curl your weights in the direction of your shoulder. Roll the ball and weights back to their starting position over the count of 8. Attempt as many as eight reps before changing legs and repeating.

Hip Twist

This exercise targets your core, outer hips and glutes. Lie on the ball with your right side over it, extending your legs and placing your right palm on the floor. Your weight should balance on the outside of your right foot and your right hand.

Put your left leg directly over the right one, and put your left hand on your hip. Raise the left leg so it is parallel with your hip height. At the top, rotate your leg while turning your toes up.

Keep the leg rotated as you lower back down over the count of 8. Turn your leg back to its starting position. Make your goal a dozen reps before switching sides and repeating the movements.

All of these movements, taken together in an exercise regimen, contribute to increasing your resting metabolic rate (RMR). This refers to the number of calories you burn before you add in activity or about two thirds of the calories you burn each day.

If you know this number, you have a good idea of the amount of food and exercise you need each day. If you can get to the point of exercising at least half an hour, five days a week, you will be well on your way toward building your metabolism to the point where weight loss can occur rapidly.

6: Foods That Make You Lose Weight Quickly

Here's the deal: when it comes to losing weight, you have to burn more calories that you take in. This means that diet is one of the main factors for dropping pounds. If you can change your dietary habits a little bit, you can lose weight much more efficiently. Why? In general terms, foods that are high in carbs have more calories but are ultimately less filling.

That's why you're going to be hungry an hour after you've had two or three donuts, but if you'd eaten the same number of calories of eggs and sausage, you would still feel full. Protein-rich foods stay with you longer than carb-rich ones. That's just one of the principles at work in this chapter. Take a look at these foods that will help you drop the weight.

1. Nuts

Are you driving around town running errands when you feel some of your biggest snack urges? Instead of pulling into the drive through and getting an unhealthy meal, reach into the console for that can of nuts. Whether its pecans, walnuts, almonds or peanuts, a handful or two can stop the cravings, and the protein keeps you full longer.

2. Dark Chocolate

Dieting doesn't mean saying "No" to your favorite flavors. However, instead of baking brownies get yourself a couple of squares of dark chocolate. The calorie count is quite low, and studies show that people who eat dark chocolate will eat a smaller meal a few hours later.

3. Soup

When you sit down to eat, have a cup of soup first. No matter whether the soup is all pureed or has chunks in it, as long as it has a broth base, you are likely to eat less with your main meal. Stay away from soups with creamy bases, and keep the calorie count at no more than 150 per serving. You'll find yourself eating less and losing weight.

4. Beans

Protein is an important part of a weight loss diet; because it keeps you full longer than carbs do. Beans are cheap to buy and work well in a number of different dishes. The fact that they take a while to digest and contain a lot of fiber keeps you feeling like you are full longer and eating less.

5. Apples

This doesn't mean apple juice or applesauce. Instead, pick up an apple and eat it. When you eat whole fruit, your appetite is controlled more effectively than when you use sauces or juices. The fruit itself has a lot more fiber, and the chewing action tells your brain that you've taken in some substantial nutrients.

6. Pureed vegetables

Let's face it - most people don't like vegetables, and adding them to a weight loss program seems like added torture to many. However, if you puree them and add them to your favorite foods, you're more likely to eat them. One popular trick is to puree some zucchini or cauliflower and add it to a bowl of macaroni and cheese.

You'll end up taking in fewer calories, because you'll think you ate a normal bowl of cheesy goodness, but the vegetables in what you ate have fewer carbs.

7. Mushrooms

Studies have shown that people who eat entrees based on mushrooms; they come away feeling just as full as when they had eaten the same entrees with beef. Mushrooms have a small fraction of the fat and calories of even the leanest cuts of beef, so making this swap can help your diet out considerably.

8. Eggs

No, we're not talking about egg whites. Eggs are a superfood for losing weight, because they help you feel full all day long. Studies show that people who have eggs with their breakfast feel full longer and lose more than double the weight as those who get their calories from a bagel. You don't have to connect eggs with breakfast either; there are many ways to incorporate them into your lunch and dinner plans.

9. Low Calorie Desserts

These aren't always the healthiest snacks, but let's face it - sometimes your body will just shout out for indulgence. A study in the Proceedings of the National Academy of Sciences shows that if you simply ban all sugary foods from your diet, you are more likely to end up overeating. It turns out that when you cut out your access to sweet foods, your brain releases a substance called corticotrophin-releasing factor (CRF), which is a response to anxiety, fear or stress. When your stress level goes up, you're likely to binge on non-nutritious foods. So unwrap one of those 100-calorie treats instead of going for the full-calorie version.

10. Oatmeal

Some carbohydrates enter the system faster than others, and the "slow releasing" ones in oatmeal and bran-based cereals can help you burn fat in some cases, particularly if you exercise after breakfast. These carbs don't send your blood sugar spiking as quickly as refined carbs, such as those you'll find in doughnuts or white bread. As a result, your insulin doesn't jump as high. Insulin is what tells your body to hoard fat, so when you have lower insulin levels, you don't keep as much fast on hand.

11. Hot Chile Peppers

Studies have shown that just adding a little bit of hot pepper a half hour before you eat helps you eat about 10 percent less. If you doubt this, go to a pizza buffet and take a look at the toppings. Often, the cooks will add onion or jalapeno to the pizza. The reason for this is that consumers will eat less pizza with that spicy intake. Less pizza eaten means more profits for the restaurant owners.

Print this list out and take it with you the next time you go to the grocery store. While you can't put together a full week's menu from it, it does give you some important principles to bear in mind when you're preparing meals. Adding some or all of these to what you eat will bring positive results within a week or two. Don't forget to keep exercising, so that you are still burning as many calories as possible.

7: Meals to Boost Your Metabolism

Do you find yourself sagging around 2 or 3 in the afternoon? Or are you tempted by the contents of your pantry after 11:00 at night? You might be one of those people who hit the ground running when you wake up in the morning, but it's likely that you have one or more points in the day when your energy level hits a low point.

If you're tired of this metabolic roller coaster, the best way to climb off is to eat at the right time and in the right amount so that your energy levels remain constant. This will help you keep your weight manageable, stay in a positive frame of mind and minimize those cravings.

It's all about portion control, nutrient mixture and the timing of when you eat. This gives you energy all day long, so that you're not riding that mental and physical roller coaster. Take a look at the meal guide below to get some ideas for specific options for snacks and meals. This will give you a boost without that awful crash that sugar and caffeine can give you.

Breakfast (usually between 6 and 8 in the morning)

Here are four choices:

- Whole grain cereal sprinkled with almonds and blueberries

- A pair of hard boiled eggs with a slice of whole grain toast and half a grapefruit

- Two slices of French toast

- Two egg vegetable omelet that contains a full cup of vegetables.

How does this boost your metabolism? When it's time for breakfast, it's likely that you have not eaten anything for as long as 12 hours, or even longer. Your body's metabolism is waiting for a signal to turn on and start burning fuel again. This time frame is the best window to cue your body to start the engine again. If you don't eat during (or close to) this window, your body and brain will slide into what is called "energy debt." Your metabolism will slow down, and you will feel fatigue and low energy levels.

Snack (usually between 9:30 and 10:30 in the morning)

Here are three choices:

- a large apple

- a 16 ounce fruit smoothie with a serving of whey protein powder

- a cup of yogurt with a whole grain fruit bar

How does this boost your metabolism? All of these snacks contain complex carbohydrates that take longer to digest than what you would get from a donut, pastry or even some granola bars.

A lot of the time, the mid-morning is the time for your first energy slump, because your work day has been a bear from the beginning, and your body has already burned through the calories you put into it this morning. These complex carbohydrates take longer to digest, giving you a sense of fullness and energy longer into the day.

Lunch (usually between noon and 1 in the afternoon)

Here are three choices:

- a vegetarian burger (patties are available in your grocer's freezer)
- an open faced turkey sandwich with vegetables
- a wrap with a couple slices of lean deli meat with tomatoes

How does this boost your metabolism? Lean meat is a great booster for dopamine production in the body. This substance stimulates metabolic activity and circulation. Lean meat also helps the body produce norepinephrine, which helps you feel more motivated and gives you focus.

Eating this type of food at lunchtime gives you that boost that you need to make it through the rest of your work day.

Snack (usually between 2 and 3 in the afternoon)

Here are four options:

- a couple pieces of string cheese

- a half cup of edamame
- a couple dozen almonds or walnuts

- a quarter cup of sunflower seeds

How does this boost your metabolism? The late afternoon is a time when you start slowing down your caloric consumption to prepare for the evening. Remember, you want an optimal cycling of metabolic activity throughout the day and night.

This is why simple, low-carb, high-protein snacks are the best, and it's a good idea to keep it simple. Natural foods have fewer carbs and have more dietary fiber than processed foods, taking longer to digest so that you don't feel cravings a few hours later.

Dinner (usually between 5:30 and 6:30 in the evening)

Here are three options:

- a cup of cremini mushrooms, 10 spears of roasted asparagus, and a half cup of brown rice;

- a chicken and spinach enchilada

- a grilled shrimp salad with walnuts and pears

How does this boost your metabolism? Now that you're about to enter the time of day when you need the least energy, get your carbs from vegetables, and maximize your protein.

These types of foods are the easiest on your blood sugar levels, so your body won't have to release as much insulin to manage what you've eaten. This helps your body get ready for the most efficient metabolism during your period of sleep.

Dessert (no less than 2 hours before you go to bed)

Here are three options:

- 1 fruit smoothie popsicle

- 1 slice of banana protein bread (put protein powder in when you bake it)

- a cup of yogurt with fresh blackberries

How does this boost your metabolism? As you are sleeping, your body is either burning fat or storing it away. Maximize the fat burn by keeping refined sugars out of your diet at dessert time. Make your dessert from complex carbohydrates, either from dairy products that are low in fat, whole grains or a smoothie. You'll sleep more soundly, and your body will burn calories and fat more efficiently. When you wake up, your mind will be clearer.

Obviously, these recipes just represent the tip of the iceberg when it comes to revving up your metabolism. Most of these ideas are simple to execute, which is important when you're talking about making major nutritional changes in your life.

Use this list of ideas to put together your next grocery list, and shop for the ingredients for the items that you think will be the most delicious. After all, dieting already represents enough of a change for most people, so you want the change to be as pleasant as possible.

8: Recipes for a Faster Metabolism

It is not easy to lose weight, and keeping that weight off can be even more difficult. However, there are some easy diet strategies that you can use along the way. Most of these diets centers around a few basic principles, such as eating a lot of dietary fiber and protein, and keeping the carbs that you eat healthy. This keeps your metabolism on more of an even keel, so that you feel like you are full for the entire day.

If you don't know how to get those principles into your daily diet, you are far from alone. Many people struggle to get their diet to a place where it is convenient enough for them on a regular basis. Take a look at the recipes in this chapter to get a sense of how you can start making this transformation in the way that you eat.

Feta and Broccoli Omelet with Toast

Want a protein charged breakfast to start your day? Not only do the egg and feta combine to give your metabolism a boost that will help you feel full until lunch, but the broccoli also is high in calcium, a nutrient that has been shown to speed up your metabolism. The whole grain toast is slower to digest than bread made from refined carbs, helping the energy to stay with you longer.

Preparation Time:

Five minutes Cooking Time:

Ten minutes Yield:

One serving

Calories per serving: 390 Fat per serving: 19g (6g saturated fat, 5g monounsaturated fat, 2g polyunsaturated fat)

Protein per serving: 23g Carbs per serving: 35g Fiber per serving: 6g Cholesterol per serving: 440mg Sodium per serving

Ingredients:

- 1 cup broccoli

- Chopped 2 large eggs beaten

- 2 slices whole grain bread

- toasted1/4 teaspoon dill dried

- 2 tablespoons feta cheese, crumbled

Place a nonstick skillet over medium heat. Coat the skillet with cooking spray. Add the broccoli and allow it to cook for three minutes. Then, put the feta, dill and egg into a small bowl to mix. Add the mixture to the skillet.

Cook for up to four minutes before flipping, and then cook for two more minutes or until the omelet is thoroughly cooked. Serve with the toast.

Honey Grapefruit and Banana

If you want to keep the weight off, this is a tangy fruit salad that tastes delicious while helping you meet your goals. You can serve this for breakfast or as a fun side dish with brunch or lunch. The effect that grapefruit has on your production of insulin makes it one of the optimal foods for helping you lose weight.

Also, grapefruit has a way to make you feel full longer because of its high water concentration (almost 90 percent of a grapefruit's weight comes from water). That juice helps you feel full so you don't overeat.

Preparation:
Five minutes Yield:
Three servings (one cup each)
Calories per serving: 122
Fats per serving: 0.4g (0.1 saturated fat, negligible amount of monounsaturated and polyunsaturated fats)
Protein per serving:
1.5g carbs per serving: 31.3gFiber per serving:
3.4g cholesterol per serving:
0g Iron per serving:
0.6mg sodium per serving:
2mg calcium per serving: 26mg
Ingredients:

- 1 banana sliced

- 1 tablespoon honey

- 24 ounces red grapefruit sections (approximately two cups

- 1 tablespoon fresh mint, chopped

Drain the sections of grapefruit, but reserve a quarter cup of juice. Mix the juice, sections and other ingredients in a medium bowl. Toss the mixture gently to provide an even coating. Serve right away, or cover and place in the refrigerator to chill.

Barbecue Turkey Burgers

Everyone loves hamburgers, but the excess fat that is often in beef can make it a no-no for dieters. However, if you are looking to minimize your beef consumption and go to a higher percentage of turkey, this is a great way. You'll be eating a great lean protein instead. Lean proteins help you feel like you're full for a longer period of time, and they contain the amino acids that you need to build muscle mass - while also speeds up your metabolism.

Yield: Four burgers

Calories per serving: 324 Fat per serving:

11g (2.7g saturated fat, 3.3g monounsaturated fat

3.9 polyunsaturated fat) Protein per serving:

28g carbs per serving:

28g fiber per serving:

1g cholesterol per serving:

75mg Iron per serving:

3mg sodium per serving:

387mg calcium per serving: 71mg

Ingredients:

1 pound dark meat turkey ground

1/2 teaspoon paprika

1/4 teaspoon ground cumin Kosher

Salt to taste

1 clove garlic, minced

1/4 teaspoon black pepper, freshly ground

4 slices sweet onion, grilled

4 sesame seed buns, toasted

1/4 cup barbecue sauce

Mix the garlic, turkey, cumin and paprika in a medium bowl. Form the mixture into four patties, seasoning with pepper and salt to taste. Heat the grill to a medium-high setting. Cook about seven minutes on each side until the burgers have cooked through. Remove from the grill and serve with the buns and any toppings that you would like.

Salmon Noodle Bowl

This dish looks like you spent hours on it, but you can make it in thirty minutes. You'll find an explosion of metabolism boosters in your dinner bowl. The avocado and salmon are bursting with the healthy kind of fats, and your veggies and noodles are all high in dietary fiber. The best ingredient from a nutritional standpoint is the asparagus, giving you a spectrum of minerals and vitamins, including A and C as well as iron and folate.

Preparation time:

Eight minutes cooking time:

Twenty minutes Yield:

Two servings Calories per serving:

492 fat per serving: 21.9g (3g saturated, 10g monounsaturated and 6.4g polyunsaturated fats)

Protein per serving:

29g carbs per serving: 47g fiber per serving:

7g cholesterol per serving: 54mg iron per serving:

3mg sodium per serving: 783mg calcium per serving: 58mg

Ingredients:

5 ounces asparagus, sliced into thirds

4 ounces whole wheat spaghetti or soba buckwheat noodles

6 ounce salmon fillet, sliced into eight pieces

1 tablespoon sesame oil, toasted

3 tablespoons lime juice

Salt and fresh pepper to taste

4 ounces cucumber (skin on), sliced into medium pieces

1/2 small avocado, cut into bite size pieces

Boil water in a pot, and then cook the noodles until they are soft (about eight minutes for spaghetti but only six for the soba noodles). Move the pasta to a strainer with tongs. Add asparagus to that same pot of boiling water. Cook for a couple of minutes, until the asparagus is ready al dente. Then rinse the asparagus under cold water.

Put a skillet on the stove at medium high heat. Coat it with cooking spray. Cook your salmon here for about three minutes on each side, to cook the middle thoroughly. Whisk the lime juice and zest, sesame oil and pepper and salt in a small bowl. Mix this dressing along with the noodles and asparagus in a larger serving bowl. Finally, add the avocado and cucumber, tossing the whole mixture to coat. Add the salmon right before you serve. Serve the salad while the salmon is still warm.

9: 7 Healthy Rules to Burn Fat

When people think about losing weight, one of the first places they look is right down at their bellies. This is a good thing, because the fat that gathers at the belly has the most harmful effects on the body. Not only does a big waist look unattractive, but those lines are symptoms of a number of possible medical problems.

You might think that the best way to target fat around the abdomen is by doing crunches or sit-ups. It's true that all exercise is helpful, but fat in that part of the body comes from excess levels of cortisol, a hormone that our body releases when we are going through stress. Cortisol breaks down the lean muscle in the body (the tissue that consumes calories with the highest efficiency) and tells the abdomen to store fat.

If you are stressing out about losing weight, the cortisol your body is producing may be counteracting the good work you are doing. Put these ten tips to work for you when it comes to burning fat.

1. *Get enough sleep*

When you don't get the right amount of sleep, you eat more food. Tired bodies produce greater amounts of ghrelin, a hormone that causes you to crave sugars and other foods that lead to the storage of fat. If you don't get enough sleep, those cortisol levels can change so that your body stores more fat as a response to insulin. Aim for at least seven hours of sleep each night if you want to achieve maximum fitness and fat burning.

1. *Exercise in intervals*

You might think that going for a three-mile jog is going to give you all of the results that you want. While jogging is good, exercising at a lower intensity level like that is not enough when it comes to burning fat. Instead, you need to use shorter, more intense bursts. The same goes for crunches: even if you did 500 a day, you wouldn't burn fat at a high rate, and your belly would actually get bigger, because the fat would have stronger muscles underneath.

Instead of jogging three miles alternate between jogging and sprinting. Instead of just doing crunches do exercises that involve all of the muscle groups in your body. Also, interrupt your work day by taking several walking breaks.

1. Stay away from sugar

Torching fat off your body is mostly a function of what you eat. Instead of eating mostly carbs, fill your plate with whole grains, vegetables and proteins. Go to the cupboard, throw out the junk food snacks, and replace them with healthy ones.

When you do crave a sweet taste, make the right substitution. Instead of running out for that high calorie latte, drink something like a lite Muscle Milk instead. There is no sugar, but the sweet taste of the chocolate flavoring will make you think there is. Also, using cinnamon instead of sugar as a sweetener makes a big difference, as cinnamon has shown in studies that it can stabilize sugar levels. Cinnamon also slows digestion, so that you feel full longer after eating.

1. Add fat to your plate

Add fat? That might seem counterintuitive, but the truth is that if you want to burn fat, you have to consume fat. It's sugar consumption that leads to the development of fat in the body, rather than the consumption of fat. This doesn't mean that you need to cut the fat off your steak and eat it whole, though. Instead, you need to pursue healthy fats, those high in Omega 3 fatty acids.

Salmon, walnuts and avocado are all relatively high in fat, but it is the healthy fat. Also, the protein that you get from these foods will help keep you full all day long.

1. Don't forget your Vitamin C

Remember cortisol, that stress hormone? Vitamin C is your tool to fight spikes in cortisol, as it balances the amount of this hormone in the body. Vitamin C helps your body create carnitine, a substance that your body uses to convert fat into a type of fuel.

In other words, Vitamin C helps you burn fat. If you find yourself going through a tough time emotionally, or through a lot of stress on the job, boost your Vitamin C consumption. It will fight the harmful side effects of all that excess cortisol. This means eating more oranges, kiwi, kale and bell peppers.

1. Don't breathe

OK, you can't stop breathing without having some very serious health complications. However, you can slow your breathing down. If you find yourself feeling tense about something, take a moment to monitor your breathing. When people undergo stress, they either breathe rapidly, with shallow breaths, or they alternate breathing quickly with holding their breath.

Once you sense the changes in your own breathing, make an effort to relax your abdomen and bring your breathing rate down. This cuts your bodily reaction to stress, which means that you will be producing less cortisol (and developing less belly fat).

1. Add to your protein consumption

If you want your body to keep lean muscle, you need to eat food with protein. If you are doing strength training, you need at least twice as much as the recommended daily allowance of protein, because your exercise is torching what you are taking in. To make it easy, try to eat a gram of protein for every pound of body weight that you have.

10: Which Supplements Should You Use?

It's great that you've decided to shed some pounds. You're joining a quest that millions just like you have started. Unfortunately, far too many people who are committed to losing weight end up failing. They start out by dropping a few pounds in water weight, only to have the weight return a few weeks later.

Changing a nutritional regimen is often more difficult than people can handle and committing to an exercise plan also represents a major life change. This is the reason for the full parking lots around health clubs and recreation centers in the evenings in January and February, right after people make New Year's resolutions to lose weight and get in shape. By March or April, though, only the diehards are left.

Losing weight involves a simple formula: if you burn more calories than you consume, you will lose weight. If you don't, then you won't. There are some pills that come with claims that they will help your metabolism shoot up in intensity, so that you will simply drop pounds.

However, these supplements are usually expensive, and even when they do work, if you stop taking the pills, the weight comes back. There are no long-term ways to get around the simple formula of calories in versus calories out.

With that said, there are some nutritional supplements that you can add to your diet. These aren't the bottles of pills that promise sudden weight loss, though. These are supplement forms of nutrients that are in the foods that we eat. If you're not getting enough of them in your diet, then you need to start adding these supplements to your daily eating plan so that you get the most benefit out of your diet.

Vitamin C

If you enjoy eating fruit, particularly the citrus variety, then you probably get enough Vitamin C in your diet. If you don't eat a lot of fruit, or it's that time of year when these fruits are not in season, then adding a C supplement (or just a simple multivitamin) can make a lot of difference. When you have stress, your body produces a hormone called cortisol. This tells your body to store fat where you probably want it the least - in your abdominal area.

Vitamin C helps to fight the production of cortisol. If you are getting the right amount of C and managing your stress level correctly, then cortisol won't be giving you that big belly that you don't want.

Calcium

Many different studies have shown that calcium helps to boost your metabolism and helps you lose weight as well. Not everyone likes to drink milk, though, and some calcium sources, like ice cream, come with too many carbs and fats to be a viable primary vehicle.

If you don't get enough calcium through your diet, adding a calcium pill to your regimen makes sense. Not only will you have stronger bones, but you will also have a metabolism that operates at a more vibrant speed, burning calories more efficiently.

Caffeine

One thing that you will read time and time again about weight loss is the importance of cutting sodas out of your diet, whether they are regular (sweetened with sugar or corn syrup) or calorie-free. However, the caffeine that is in soda is not a source of concern, at least not in terms of weight loss.

In fact, caffeine is one of the best sources of a metabolism boost that you can get. Whether it's through coffee, tea (or even soda), caffeine is one of the world's most common substances when it comes to getting a boost of energy, either in the morning or afternoon.

A study at the University of Maryland Medical Center indicates that there may be a strong connection between caffeine and green tea; taken together, they may be able to help your body burn more fat at the cellular level. However, you will want to talk to your physician before you decide to use caffeine to speed up your metabolism.

Whey Protein Powder

Smoothies are a great way to get those servings of fruit and vegetables without having to choke down those green foods that you just don't like to eat. You can put spinach or broccoli into a blender with some fruits and end up with a smoothie that tastes much better than either of those two vegetables. You can add a serving of whey protein powder to amp up your results even more.

Soy protein also comes in powder form, but studies have shown that soy protein amps up your levels of estrogen. Especially for guys, this is not something you want to happen, because that erodes your levels of testosterone, which helps you do everything from build muscle to act assertively to achieve strong erections in the bedroom.

Whey protein does not affect the sexual hormones, but instead contributes to both muscle mass and higher metabolism. Adding a serving to your smoothies will super charge your diet.

Fish Oil

There are good fats and there are bad fats. The fats that you slice off your steak, that's the bad kind. The fats that's inside a grilled salmon, that's the good kind. It's rich in Omega-3 fatty acids, which help your body build up the "good" cholesterol (the HDL kind).

However, not everyone is going to get a serving of fish each day, even though studies show that's a great thing to do in your diet if you want to stay trim. This is where fish oil supplements come in. These pills contain the healthy fatty acids that you need in order to drop weight and keep it off, but you don't have to actually eat the fish. Not everyone is a big fan of seafood, and others only like fish when it's fried (which counteracts the good of the fish oil inside). So add a fish oil pill to your nutritional regimen, and you'll like the results.

None of these supplements will replace the good that a combination of healthy eating and rigorous, regular exercise will produce for the body. However, if you are already on a positive path with diet and exercise, these supplements can make your progress go even more quickly.

Make it easy, try to eat a gram of protein for every pound of body weight that you have. One easy way to do this is to add a serving of protein, such as eight ounces of low-fat yogurt, two tablespoons of nuts or three ounces of lean meat to each snack or meal. Over the course of your day, this will give you the protein you need.

If you can make these changes, you will start to see results in a matter of weeks. You'll feel better, and you'll notice that your clothes fit better, because that unwanted fat is going away, and you're returning to your ideal shape.

Conclusion

Hopefully this book has helped you find some new strategies for managing your diet and putting together an exercise plan that will help you lead to a long-term, sustained weight loss. There are few things more frustrating than dropping those first eight or ten pounds, only to see them show up again on the scale.

It's important to remember that you are not alone on your quest for health. If you have the funds, join a gym in your neighborhood. You'll meet people who have the same interests that you have. Most gyms offer a free evaluation with a trainer, which means that you can get a list of suggested workouts without spending any more money.

Many cities have running clubs that form at local running stores. If the idea of jogging or running seems beyond you, many of these clubs split their workouts into different pace groups, including a group of walkers. Runners are friendly people, so if you do not have any physical limitations that would keep you from walking, this is a great way to start your fitness journey.

As far as your trips to the grocery store, the easiest way to make a start is to stick to the "U" - Only take your cart around the outside walls of the store. You'll find meat, produce and dairy - natural foods that don't have the refined sugars of processed foods. Your journey toward nutritional health will be a long one, but you will enjoy the changes you undergo along the way.

12715228R00045

Printed in Great Britain
by Amazon.co.uk, Ltd.,
Marston Gate.